# The Mystery of Health is Wealth

## By Precious David

# Table of Content

# CHAPTER 1

**INTRODUCTION**

Good Health is the wish of God to all Christians according to 3 John 2 "Beloved, I beg that you flourish in all things and health, just as your soul prospers". Health is a measure of riches because neither the dead nor the ill can worship God (Psalm 115:17). (Psalm 115:17). We are God's handiwork created in Christ Jesus for good works, which God planned that we should walk in them (Eph 2:70). (Eph 2:70). He wants us to work hard and contribute to the kingdom's progress.

The saying 'health is wealth' indicates a condition of well-being free from disease(s), whether physically or emotionally. The proverb is an old one, as may be noticed from a renowned antique Rome poet, Virgil "The greatest treasure is Health" Virgil is supposed to have experienced ill health throughout his life, and possibly it is probable that the condition of his health motivated him to propose this aphorism as words of counsel for the following generation.


Some proven adages/quotes stating health is wealth are as follows: It's health that is actual riches and not bits of Gold and silver (Gandhi) (Gandhi). So many spend their cash to reclaim their health (A. J Materiri) (A. J Materiri). "Health is priceless wealth. Invest while you can." Bryant McGill

## HEALTH DEFINITION

HEALTH is a state of complete physical, mental, and social well-being and not merely the absence of diseases (WHO) (WHO). Physical is the body. Mental is about how individuals think and feel. Social welfare is about how individuals connect.

## GENERAL FACTORS THAT COULD AFFECT YOUR HEALTH

1. Belief system: Some believe that seeking medical attention depicts a lack of faith in God but scripturally speaking it is not true (Luke 5:31, Jeremiah 8:22).

2. Lack of time for health-promoting activities such as (a) Skipping breakfast just to catch up with work time.

(b) Skipping morning prayer and praises to catch up with work time (Proverb 3:6-8). (Proverb 3:6-8).

(c) Skipping early workouts only to catch up with work time.

3. Laziness combined with urbanization is making many of us depend on fast food (junk food) on a daily basis.

4. Limited resources in a harsh economy is a big factor affecting our attention to our health, especially going to hospitals.

5. Introduction of Supplements / Quacks in the market space has made many people feel relaxed about seeking proper medical care.

6. Lack of priority to our health has made many people not see the need to get personal first aid machines such as BP machines, Glucometer, and BMI.

7. Depending on social media information.

8. Depending on self-treatment and previous knowledge.

9. Depending on information from neighbors and friends who are not medical experts.

10. Poor hygiene system is harmful to health:

(a) Less attention to regular hand washing enhances the spread of communicable diseases e.g Covid-19, Cholera, TB, etc.

(b) Untidy environment is the breeding ground for mosquitoes, malaria is preventable if we perform the essentials.

(c) Sharing of barbing clippers with the public.

(d) Sharing of a drinking cup with the public e.g the usage of a single drinking cup by youngsters in the church is not recommended.

(e) Improper flushing of toilet before and after use.

(f) Washing of hands after toilet without medicated soap.

11. Poor dietary system is harmful to health:

(a) Deficiency of Vitamin A in the body causes night blindness, of course, it is only gotten from the meal we eat daily.

(b) Lack of a balanced diet predisposes many to diabetes.

(c) Lack of a balanced diet predisposes many to cancer.

(d) Lack of a balanced diet predisposes many to hypertension.

(e) Lack of a balanced diet predisposes many to obesity.

## SOME TRENDING HEALTH ISSUES

Eye Health

"The eye is the candle of the body. If your eyes are healthy your entire body will be full of light" (Mathew 6:22 NIV) (Mathew 6:22 NIV). It consequently suggests that a healthy eye is a healthy body. The eye is the diagnostic hub of the body. An eye expert may identify disorders of the body such as hypertension or diabetes through a basic eye examination. An eye specialist provides a remedy to other health difficulties of the body owing to his/her important involvement in systemic disorders identification. My brothers, I want to call our attention to the hazard of regular eye rubbing.

It is extremely essential to realize that eye rubbing (scratching) as a consequence of irritation is risky for the following reasons:

1. The eye can never get better during rubbing; instead it will become red and swollen more.

2. During rubbing more infections are introduced into the eye.

3. During rubbing you could damage the cornea, once it happens, blindness sets in immediately. The cornea is the window of the eye, the cornea is comparable to the exterior windscreen of a vehicle, if the windscreen is damaged the driver's eyesight will be impacted, similar to if the cornea is damaged in the course of eye rubbing the person's vision will be damaged.

4. Eye rubbing could cause many eye diseases like trichiasis, ulcer, etc. If you

attentively watch you will notice individuals having ball-like growth on their eyelids, this is due to eye rubbing. The ball-like is primarily prevalent among youngsters who routinely perform eye rubbing.

We must thus put a halt to excessive eye rubbing if we wish to enjoy good vision: You may prefer to place little pressure on your closed eyelids instead of massaging them.

## MATERNAL HEALTH

Maternal Health refers to the health of women throughout pregnancy, delivery, and the postnatal period (WHO) (WHO).

The most prevalent direct causes of maternal injury and death are:

1. Severe bleeding (mostly bleeding after childbirth) (mostly bleeding after childbirth).

2. Infection (usually after birth) (usually after birth).

3. High blood pressure during pregnancy (pre-eclampsia and eclampsia) (pre-eclampsia and eclampsia).

4. Complication from delivery (Labour) (Labour).

5. Unsafe abortion.

6. Other causes are associated with infections such as malaria or related chronic conditions like cardiac diseases and diabetes.

**The main factors that prevent women from receiving or seeking care during pregnancy and childbirth are:**

1. Poverty.

2. Distance to facilities.

3. Lack of information.

4. Inadequate and poor quality services.

5. Cultural beliefs and practices.

## THE CHURCH ROLES IN MATERNAL HEALTH

1. The church should not only pray for the pregnant members but should also encourage them to go for antenatal care at the nearest Government approved Health facilities.

2. The church should encourage its members to seek professional pieces of advice on family planning to avoid unprepared pregnancy.

## HYPERTENSIVE HEART DISEASES

It refers to the cardiac issues induced by excessive blood pressure. The heart functioning under increasing strain produces cardiac diseases. My nice suggestion to everyone is easy, simply go to the local health clinic and check your BP periodically. It will rescue you from abrupt death owing to hypertensive heart conditions.

**RISKS OF HYPERTENSIVE HEART DISEASES**

High blood pressure (Hypertension) is the number one danger, and the risk rises with the following:

1. Overweight.

2. No proper exercise.

3. Smoking.

4. Eating food high in fat and cholesterol.

5. Stress.

**HYPERTENSION PREVENTION**

1. Reduce salt to less than 5g daily.

2. Eat fruit and vegetables regularly.

3. Avoid saturated fats and trans fat.

4. Avoid tobacco.

5. Reduce alcohol.

6. Be physically active every day.

7. Check your BP routinely.

8. Proper stress management.

9. Check your Fasting Blood Sugar (FBS) routinely.


**STRESS AND MANAGEMENT TIPS**

**INTRODUCTION**

Stress is the brain and body's reaction to any demand which might be physical (e.g. pushing a malfunctioning car), emotional stress (broken marriages), and biological stress (road accident) (road accident).

When the brain perceives stress in the environment, the stress response system gets into action. The stress response system of the brain includes the Amygdala, hypothalamus, pituitary gland, Adrenal gland, cortisol, and prefrontal cortex. The amygdala is positioned in the center of the brain. It is the brain structure that senses stress and notifies the HPA Axis (hypothalamus-pituitary-adrenal axis) to respond. The hypothalamus must wake up the pituitary gland. The pituitary release hormone that travels out of the brain to the adrenal gland. The adrenal gland resides on top of the kidney, and the adrenal gland produces cortisol in the body (bloodstream) (bloodstream). Cortisol urges the body into action to battle stress. The prefrontal cortex positioned in the front of the brain governs the emotional reactions to stress.

In summary, the brain response enables the body to cope with the condition creating stress. This is only the body's method of defending itself against harm. There is a long exposure to stress and the body keeps vigilant even when there is no threat. Over time, this placed the body in danger of health issues such as heart disease, asthma, obesity, diabetes, headache, depression, gastrointestinal trouble, Alzheimer's disease, accelerated aging, early mortality, forgetfulness, and hypertension.

**MANAGEMENT TIPS**

1. Identify the sources of stress in your life.

2. Make time for fun and relaxation.

3. Maintain balance with a healthy lifestyle.

4. Accept that there are events that you cannot control.

5. Learn to say no to requests that would create excessive stress in your life.

6. Get enough rest and sleep, your body needs time to recover from a stressful event.

7. Seek treatment with a psychologist or other mental health professional trained in stress management.

8. Don't rely on alcohol, drugs, or compulsive behaviors to reduce stress.

9. Keep a positive attitude.

10. Eat healthy, well-balanced meals.

11. Be conscious to know that prolonged exposure to stressors is dangerous.


**CONCLUSION**

At this point, I desire to end with this saying "information is the best prescription", the knowledge about your health told thus far is adequate for a healthy life. May God grant us the grace to remember and implement the teachings to the glory of His name. Amen.

# CHAPTER 2

## WEALTH DEFINITION

Wealth is anything that could be owned and controlled, and have monetary value or the potential to create monetary value. Wealth by dictionary definition is the abundance of valuable financial assets or physical possessions that can be converted into a form that can be used for transactions. Wealth can be either tangible or intangible or both. When we talk about a wealth of experience it is an intangible wealth. Physical cash at hand or cash in the bank, and real estates are tangible wealth.

## OBJECTIVE

The objective of this part of today's indoor lecture on the subject of "Your Wealth " is aimed at reminding Christians and our visitors here present about the importance of wealth, its sources, its creation, and its preservation for our overall well-being and sustenance. It is very important to note that Wealth is subject to Health. Ralph Waldo Emerson stated that "The First Wealth is Health ", permit me to refine that assertion and state that "The First Wealth is God" because God is the one who gives us strength to make wealth (Deut. 8:18). The richest man that ever lived – King Solomon – was granted riches, wealth and honor by God Almighty (2 Chro. 1:11, 12). The scriptures state that "Silver and gold belong to God" and that "For every beast of the forest is Mine. And the cattle on a thousand hills" (Hag. 2:8; Psa. 50:10).

Whereas wealth gets accumulated by hard work and perseverance, health which is given by God gets accumulated and improved by discipline and cleanliness; hygiene contributes to health, and earnings contribute to wealth (Prov. 10:4, 12:11, 24,

27, 13:4, 14:24, 3:7-8). One of the greatest differences between health and wealth is that wealth can be stolen and robbed by an external aggressor, however, we on our own can rob ourselves of our health by not taking care of ourselves hygienically and medically. On the other hand, we may as a result of laziness and irresponsible lifestyle push ourselves into poverty that consequently impacts our health; malnutrition, filthy living environment, inability to access quality education, etc, are indices of poverty.

It is equally important to state here that acquiring wealth, though very good, might be so engaging that we may neglect its impact on our health (physical and spiritual). Health is a state of physical, emotional, and spiritual well-being; the source of our wealth might be compromised and/or jeopardized if no attention is given to it. Indeed, health is the most important and long-lasting wealth, but unfortunately, most of us in the race to earn materialistic wealth, ignore it. If we are not healthy then we will neither be able to make more wealth nor enjoy the wealth so gathered. Interestingly, we can both create wealth or poverty depending on the choices we make. We shall, therefore, in this lecture briefly examine the scripture, and ways how to create, accumulate, preserve, utilize, and manage wealth for the overall well-being and benefit of ourselves and also for those who depend on us and look up to us for support.

**PREAMBLE**

God so loved mankind that He did not only proclaim strength to him to make wealth (Deut. 8:18), but He desired that man prosper and be in good health even as his soul prospers (3 John 2). Our Lord and Saviour Jesus Christ proclaimed in (John 10:10), that "The thief does not come except to steal, and to kill, and to destroy. I have come that they may have life and that they may have It more abundantly." This is an assurance to us of a more abundant life that encompasses total well-being of health and wealth. He also assured us of the spirit of love, power, and a sound mind (2 Tim. 1:7) "For God has not given us a spirit of fear, but of power and love and a sound mind." This embodies a sound mind in a sound body; a state of all-round well-being. Solomon in Proverbs stated; "Keep your heart with all diligence, For out of it spring the issues of life." (Prov. 4:23).

These issues of life are obvious, our physical and emotional well-being, but more importantly our spiritual health, and material wealth; desirably promoted and improved with a diligent heart. As referenced above, Sir Ralph Waldo Emerson in 1860 penned that "The first wealth is health", which I like to refine as "The first wealth is God"; because it is God that gives us the power to make wealth (Duet. 8:18). Interestingly, both health and wealth are blessings from God " Beloved, I wish above all things that you prosper and be in health, even as your soul prospers." (3 John. 2).


**DISCUSSION**

Beloved, while the first lecturer discussed "Your Health", I will briefly examine the subject of "Your Wealth". It is well known universally that physical, mental, and spiritual healthiness is the bedrock of a happy, peaceful, successful, worthy, wealthy life and living. Health is so priceless and cannot be purchased with money. You can use your health to create, make and build wealth, but it is highly difficult to use your wealth to recover and renew your health. There is this strong view that, unless a person is healthy, it is difficult for the person to enjoy wealth. Wealth does not have value unless it is enjoyed.

Simple possession of wealth (money and luxuries) does not make an individual a rich person; it is the abundance of good health. This implies that health strongly influences a person's capability to enjoy the wealth which he might have amassed or acquired. It is therefore crystal clear that above all things, the possession of health is the ultimate. An individual can be said to be healthy when his physical, mental, and spiritual well-being is at its optimum levels or gauges. Here lies happiness and pleasure.

In all these, it is also a known fact that poverty; a direct cause of lack of wealth, in itself is a disease that has a strong capacity to provoke poor health and real sickness (Prov. 6:10-11, 23:19-21, 28:19; Eccl. 6:10). Let us then examine ways of creating, accumulating, preserving, utilizing, managing wealth for our overall well-being and that of those who depend on us for support.

## WORK

It goes without saying that if we are unemployed or do not earn income, it is impossible to create or build wealth. To create wealth, we must seek to get employed or engaged in income-generating activities; starting with the primary intangible wealth or asset – the strength or power is given by God (Deut. 8:17,18). Generating surplus income requires that we struggle hard to earn an income that surpasses our basic family upkeep; a shortfall of which will mean that our potential to create wealth will be zero!

So we have only one option; increase our disposable income by (1) working much harder (1 Thess. 4:11; 1 Tim. 5:8; 2 Thess. 3:11-12), (2) looking for other honest ways of improving our income by investing (3) change our extravagant spending pattern to save money (Prov. 21:20, 29:3). Every extra Naira saved can be used to start building your wealth when applied into good income-generating assets

**SAVE**

What is money? Money is the compensation or wage received from exercising our physical and intellectual capabilities. Money when acquired answers all things, but in the same vein, the love of money is the route of all evil (Eccl. 7:12; 1Tim. 6:10). Beloved, how we make and spend our active income will have a direct influence on the amount of surplus income you will set aside for wealth creation. Do you need cable TV? What about those eating out or night out? What about those expensive attires, Jewries, Japanese/Indian hair attachments, and make-up? Are they really all necessary at this moment for you? What monthly expense can you cut out of those unnecessary excesses? Beloved, you must therefore, have a critical look at your spending patterns because surplus income determines how quickly you can start building wealth. The less you spend on things that you want (as opposed to things that you need), the more income you will have to spend on assets that will make you wealthy.

**INVEST**

Effective wealth creation is based largely on looking around us to identify and meet consumer needs and not on trying to predict business cycles. Beloved look out there in your immediate environment, there are a lot of consumer needs to fulfill. Fulfilling consumer needs is the fastest way to wealth creation. Consumer needs are very easy to identify, track and cater to, thus generating quick income.

When starting, it is not good to blow your free cash on assets that cannot produce income. Food, shelter, and clothing are basic human needs; property investment is a business because people require shelter, same for trading goods and services identified to be of need within any locality. If you supply the property and other people pay you for using it or you trade on goods and services and people pay you for them, then you are in the business of creating wealth. But be careful of Ponzi market cycles such as fixed deposits, pension funds, shares in the stock market, UMANA-UMANA, MMM, and Bitcoin; passive business investments that generate income that is exceptionally difficult to predict.

**BLOSSOM**

The secret of business sustainability and growth is largely predicated on the moral and ethical qualities as well as the integrity of the person(s) behind the business. Can people trust you with their hard-earned financial or intangible resources? Are you honest enough for people to trust you? Do you have strong moral principles? Do you respect ethical standards in your business? What is your level of integrity? (1Kgs. 9:4; Job. 27:5; Prov. 13:11, 12:1, 2, 22). Whereas morality is subjective and is measured by what is appropriate or inappropriate from a societal point of view and, in our case as children of God, strictly influenced by Christian principles, ethics on the other hand is based on an objective framework that follows an agreed code of practice in a given set of circumstances.

Christians must keep to business agreements. Please note that in business you deserve only what you negotiated, especially for those involved in "arranged" or commission agents.

We must diligently respect and avoid third-party disclosures (Prov. 11:13; 18:8; 20:19). Businesses have secrets, therefore try to acquire them, and do not steal them (1Cor. 6:10). As Christians and business owners or wealth creators, we have the moral and ethical obligation to respect business ethics, uphold moral uprightness and integrity to succeed in business and retain our faith in Christ Jesus (Lev. 19: 15-16; Deut. 25:13-15; Prov. 11:3, 20:7; 2 Cor. 8:21; Phil. 4:8; 1Thess. 4:12; 1Peter 2:12).

**GRATIFY**

With the efforts put in creating and managing wealth as outlined above, our attention should then be directed to how we will use the wealth so acquired to the glory of the source of that wealth – God Almighty and for our overall well-being. We have earlier mentioned that deferred gratification is a critical consideration in wealth accumulation, but we must at all levels of our financial growth, achievement or success determine what should be taken out to express gratitude to the source of the wealth, pamper ourselves, as well as support the needy in our midst (Deut. 16:17, 17:1, 15:7; Eccl. 3:13, 5:18; 1 Tim. 6:17-19; Gal. 6:2; 1 John 3:17).

## CONTENTMENT

In all these, we must learn to be content no matter our level of wealth acquisition. God will bless whom He will bless; do not question Him but yourself for what you have not done rightly. You must learn to be contented, do not put all your trust in your wealth (1 Tim. 6:6; 1 Tim. 6:17-19). We must learn not to be in debt; he who goes borrowing goes sorrowing (Prov. 37:21; Rom. 3:8). Use your wealth in such a way that it will bring glory to God (Jam. 4:3-4, 5:1-6).

## CONCLUSION

May God keep us prosper and be in good health even as our souls prosper in Lord Jesus Christ's Name. Amen. (3 John. 2).